THE BASIC TEN

*The Simple Way to Go from
Couch Potato to Fit*

BENJAMIN T. MUELLER

Disclaimer

You should consult your physician or other health care professional before starting this or any other fitness program, to determine if it is right for your needs. This is particularly true if you (or your family) have a history of high blood pressure or heart disease, or if you have ever experienced chest pain when exercising or have experienced chest pain in the past month when not engaged in physical activity, if you smoke, have high cholesterol, are obese, or have a bone or joint problem that could be made worse by change in physical activity. Do not start this fitness program if your physician or health care provider advises against it. If you experience faintness, dizziness, pain, or shortness of breath at any time while exercising you should stop immediately.

Contents

Introduction

Most people know the importance of exercise. Almost everyone is aware by now of the great health and mental benefits to regular physical activity. Yet so many people get caught up in the stresses of their current daily lives, they neglect to exercise.

The number-one excuse people give for not exercising is that they simply *don't have enough time.* The story for many adults goes something like this: they have to wake up early, get the kids ready for school, get dressed for work, work long hours, get dinner ready, take the kids to practice, and crash into bed, ready to do it all again the next day.

Because of this, most adults simply give up on exercise, which, unfortunately, lets their health go down the tubes. Then, every New Year, tons of people make the resolution to join a gym and exercise regularly. Unfortunately, it only takes a few weeks before people realize that, for whatever reason, they just cannot keep up with this new routine.

People need an exercise program that is simple and reliable. A program that allows them to work out regularly in less than twenty minutes, without a lot of equipment and space. Something they can do at home, in the park or a hotel room, even at the office. A program they can do wearing jeans and a T-shirt or at home in their underwear. Something they can depend on and, most importantl,y follow through with!

This book is put together in a way that is simple and easy to understand. The layout is clean, clear, and short by design. It is divided up into five parts:

1. Motivation for regular physical activity
2. Description of key exercises

3. 4-week workout program 1
4. 4-week workout program 2
5. Nutrition and recovery tips

The first section includes chapters that discuss the great mental and physical benefits of physical activity. Much of the content in these chapters may be things you already have heard of, but through this refresher, I hope it provides you clear motivation to start the simple exercise program laid out in the rest of the book.

The second section outlines and describes the ten key exercises used throughout this program. It will break down each of the core exercises and describe how to perform them safely and efficiently. It will also discuss the primary muscle groups each exercise is designed to strengthen.

The third section lays out for you the first four weeks' worth of workouts you will be performing. This will consist of a total of twenty workouts (five per week). It breaks each workout down into the exact number or reps of each individual exercise you will do for that day's workout.

The fourth section dives into the final four weeks of the program. It outlines each of those workouts, similar to the strategy in section three.

Finally, the fifth section consists of bonus content to enhance your recovery and nutrition. This is a good section to read while you are doing the workout program. Thus, it would be a good idea to bookmark the workout you are on and read past it into this fifth section as soon as you start the workout program.

Each section is further divided up into short chapters, to make it easier for you to navigate and understand the overall exercise program.

Finally, if you want to watch video demonstrations of how to perform the exercises, you can visit my Instagram video library: @TheBasicTen.

What this program will do for you?

As I said upfront, this program is designed to give you the opportunity to exercise regularly anywhere you can, including the convenience of your own home or office.

By completing this program, you will strengthen your overall muscular system and improve your cardiovascular health, as well. You will also burn a significant number of calories with each workout, which, combined with a healthy diet, can help people lose weight or maintain a healthy weight. Further improving your muscle mass will also increase your body's overall metabolism. Experts agree that a regular exercise routine such as this can decrease your risk of many diseases.

The journey you go on in undertaking this program can also boost your mental health. Research has shown that physical activity causes the brain to release chemicals called endorphins that will improve a person's mood.

The workouts should also provide a stress-reliever, as well as help people cope with overall anxiety and stress. Dr. John Ratey researched the many mental benefits of regular exercise and concluded it can reduce anxiety, improve mood, plus improve attention and overall discipline.

What this program will not do for you?

This program will not burn you out or push you over the edge like many typical exercise programs may do. That's not to say this program will not challenge you, but it does take into consideration a key fact: the body needs adequate time to recover between workouts.

Even though this workout program is an excellent way to build body strength, burn calories, and improve your metabolism, it will not promise unrealistic results. Consistency is the key to keeping yourself on track with any of your fitness goals.

This program will also not guarantee you six-pack abs or a shredded physique when you are done. If you follow the workouts and improve your diet, however, you should definitely see a better overall body composition and strength after these eight weeks.

Physical Benefits of Exercise

I'm sure you already know by now that exercise is very beneficial to your physical health. In fact, regular physical activity has been shown to reduce your risk of pretty much every disease, including the top two leading causes of death in the United States today: heart disease and cancer.

Regular physical activity also contributes to managing a healthy weight, which goes a long way to reducing your risk of disease, as well. As you exercise more and become more fit, your muscle tone and body composition will also improve. Not only is this healthier for you, overall, but it also makes you stronger and can improve your posture.

As your fitness improves, you will also find yourself with more energy throughout the day. You should find that you are more productive, going about your regular routine tasks.

Your body was designed to be active and move during each day. That said, ultimately, your body will transform into what you do to it. If you remain physically active throughout your life, all of your body systems will respond positively to that.

Mental Benefits of Exercise

Exercise is as good for your brain as it is for your body.

Some of the key mental benefits of exercise include reducing overall anxiety and stress. Physical activity will also improve your concentration and make you feel better about yourself, overall.

Many people who start an exercise program also begin to eat healthier and look out after their health in other ways.

Another great benefit of physical activity is that it has been shown to enhance a person's overall mood.

Exercise to Combat Obesity and Weight Gain

Roughly 60% of adults in developed nations are overweight, and approximately one out of every three adults is considered obese. People are simply consuming more calories than they are burning.

The number of calories you burn per workout is dependent upon your age, body size, genetics, and other factors. Let's say each workout burns an additional 200 calories per day. This means, if you do five workouts per week for four total weeks, you will burn additional 4,000 calories per month. This is slightly more than the number of calories it takes to burn off exactly one pound of body fat.

Now, if a person maintains this exercise routine for an entire year, they would weigh twelve fewer pounds after one year. Imagine what a simple exercise routine like this would do after a period of two years, five years, ten years, or more. It would definitely be the difference between being at a healthy weight versus being obese.

Optimal Workout Time and Length (Does not have to be Long)

How long does a person need to work out in order to get the mental and physical benefits of their exercise activity? This is a common question people have, after learning about the physical and mental benefits of exercise.

The answer is: not as long as you probably think! You can get enormous benefits from just ten to fifteen minutes of physical activity every day. In the last chapter, we did the math on how many calories you can burn on a monthly and yearly basis after doing just a little bit of exercise each day.

The improved brain health and other mental benefits of physical activity can be accomplished with just a simple ten-minute daily workout. In fact, shorter and faster workouts have been shown to do just as much for your health as long, slow workouts.

Research and science have shown that, after about forty-five minutes of exercise, the benefits are not as great. Simply put, a workout that lasts about fifteen to thirty minutes that includes a warm-up, a variety of exercises, and then a nice cool-down stretch is ideal.

Of course, to add to the benefits of this, you should be looking for other ways to get more physical activity, such as walking more, parking farther away from buildings, even just marching or jogging in place, doing simple exercises while watching television, and limiting the amount of sitting you're doing during the day.

Key Exercises

In the next section of this book, we are going to go through an overview of all of the key exercises included in the later workout plan. Each of these key exercises is simple and easy to perform. They can be performed at a variety of intensities, making them perfect for beginner and advanced levels. These key exercises done together will give you a full-body workout that will strengthen and tone your entire body.

It is important to perform each exercise using the correct technique. In other words, make sure you emphasize technique over speed when performing the exercises. Using the correct technique will engage your muscle groups in the most efficient way plus reduce your risk of injury.

As you read through this section, it is a good idea to practice each exercise when you finish reading about it. Also, if you go to my Instagram video library: @TheBasicTen, you will find I have posted demonstrations of each of the key exercises listed below.

Exercise 1: Jumping Jack

You probably remember doing jumping jacks as a kid. Jumping Jacks is a famous exercise used in sports to warm up both the legs and the arms. The exercise is said to have gotten its name from US General John J. "Black Jack" Pershing during World War I.

The Jumping Jack exercise is performed in the following manner:

> ➤ Start in a standing position with feet together and your hands at your side.

> ➢ Jump your feet 2-3 feet apart, straddling your legs wide, as you sweep your arms over your head so the hands touch.

> ➢ Then jump back into your starting position, feet together, arms down at your side.

> ➢ Repeat the process.

You can make Jumping Jacks more intense simply by squatting lower and jumping up as high as you can.

You can make them less intense by doing a modified version that I call "Lazy Jacks." To perform these:

> ➢ Begin by standing with feet together and arms to side (beginning position).

> ➢ Then, take a side step to the left with left leg only (keep other leg stationary) and bring your left arm up.

> ➢ Return back to the beginning position by stepping with your left leg back to meet the right and lower your left arm down to the side.

> ➢ Then repeat same process with your right side.

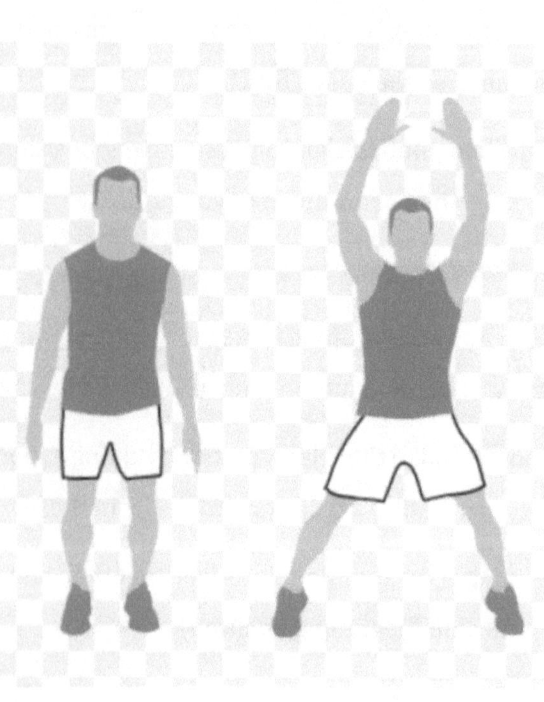

Jumping Jacks serve as a simple warm-up exercise that engages your entire body and can get your heart rate up fairly quickly.

For a video demonstration of how to perform the regular Jumping Jacks, the more intense jumping jacks, and Lazy Jacks please refer to my Instagram video library: @TheBasicTen.

Exercise 2: Squat

This squat is a simple exercise designed to engage your quadriceps, core muscles, back, and glutes. To make a squat more difficult, weight lifters generally add weight. In this program, we will not be using any weight and will just be using your own bodyweight.

To perform a squat, follow the steps below:

➢ Begin in a standing position with your legs slightly wider than your shoulders.

➢ With your feet still, lower your hips such that your knees are bent at 90 degrees and track out over your toes. Hold this position for a second or two.

➢ Then stand back up

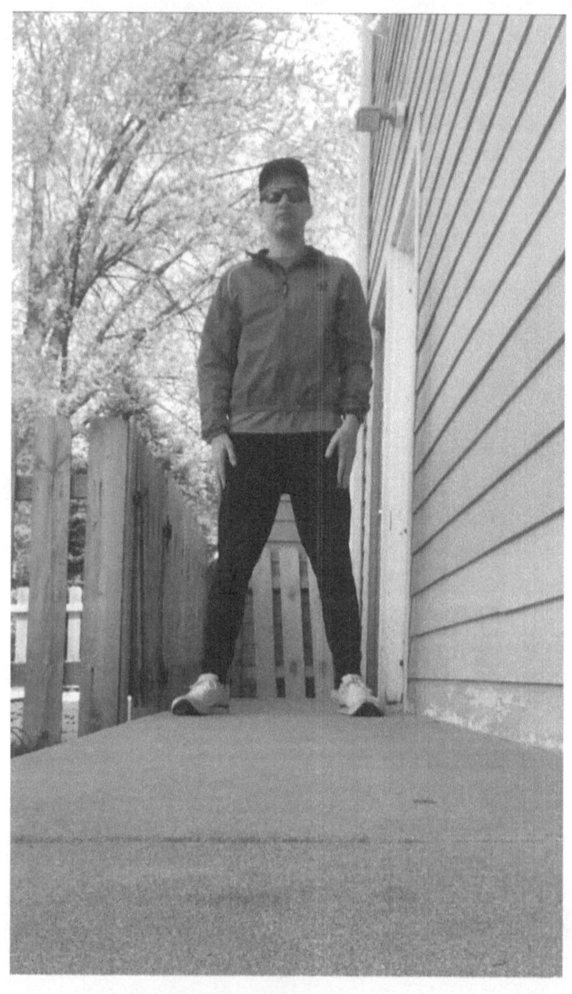

Starting position for squat.

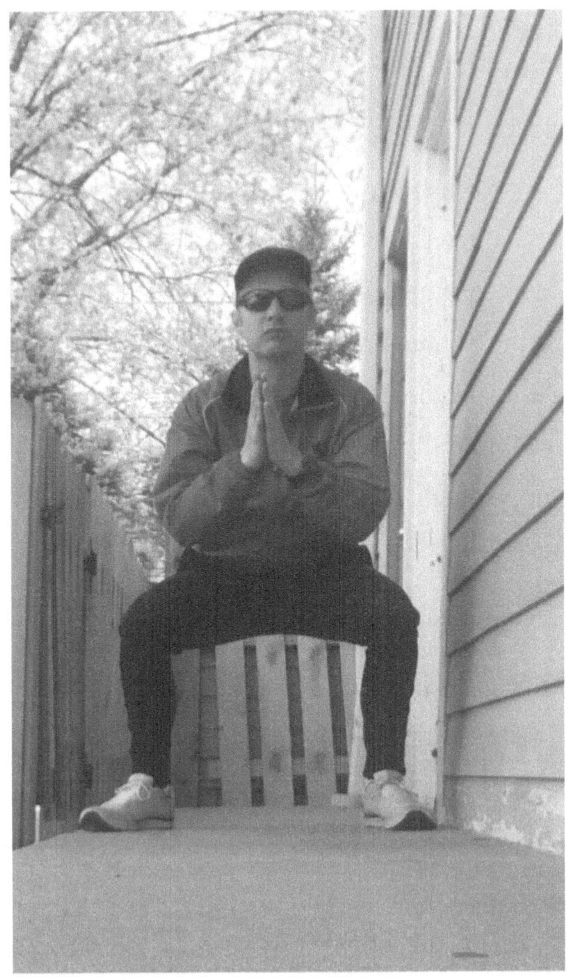

Lower until knees are bent at or close to 90 degrees.

Exercise 3: Push-up (wide, normal, and diamond)

The push-up is one of the most basic exercises to work your arms, shoulders, chest, back, and core. For those people who are new to push-ups or who do not have a lot of upper-body strength, they can begin by placing their knees on the floor and their calves and feet slightly up in the air, leaning forward ahead of your knee cap, more toward the thigh. For those who have more upper-body strength, their legs should be straight with just their toes on the floor.

The following are the steps to performing a push up:

➤ Begin with your arms slightly wider than your shoulders.

➤ Keep your chest and legs aligned as you lower your chest to the floor until it nearly touches the ground (elbows should be bent at 90 degrees).

➤ Push yourself back up to the starting position.

The key to doing a good push-up is to keep your back and legs aligned as you go down. You want to tighten your core as you lower your chest to the ground, stopping when your elbows are at 90 degrees. Also, take a deep breath in as you go down and blow the air out as you push back up.

You can change the specific types of muscles worked by making your hands wider, elbows flaring out, or do a diamond push-up, with the hands close to the center of your chest, thumb and index fingers almost touching, and elbows bending straight back, close to the sides of your ribcage.

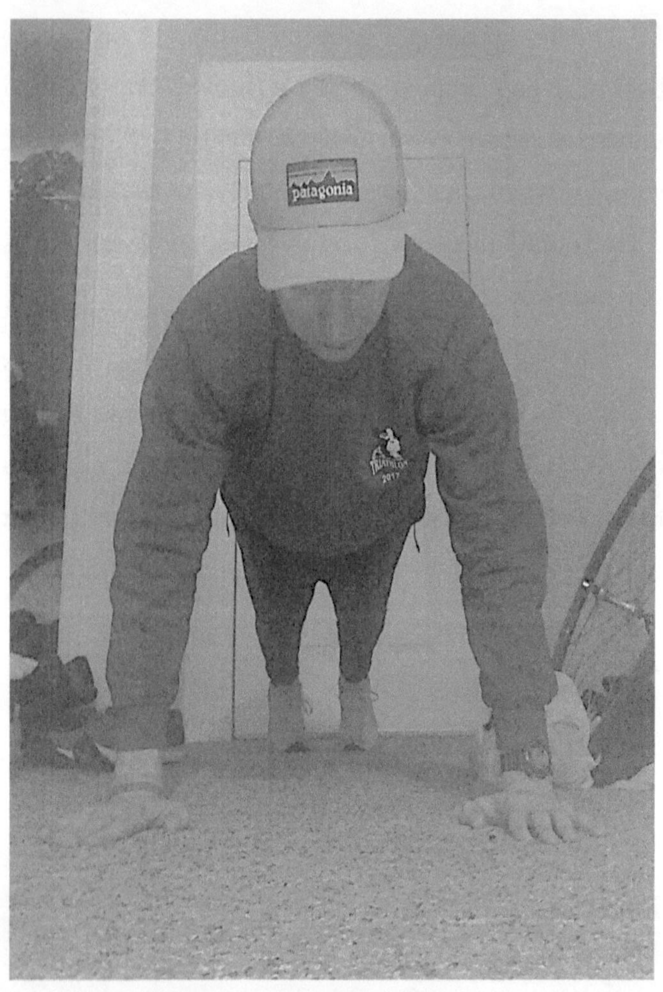

Beginning push up position

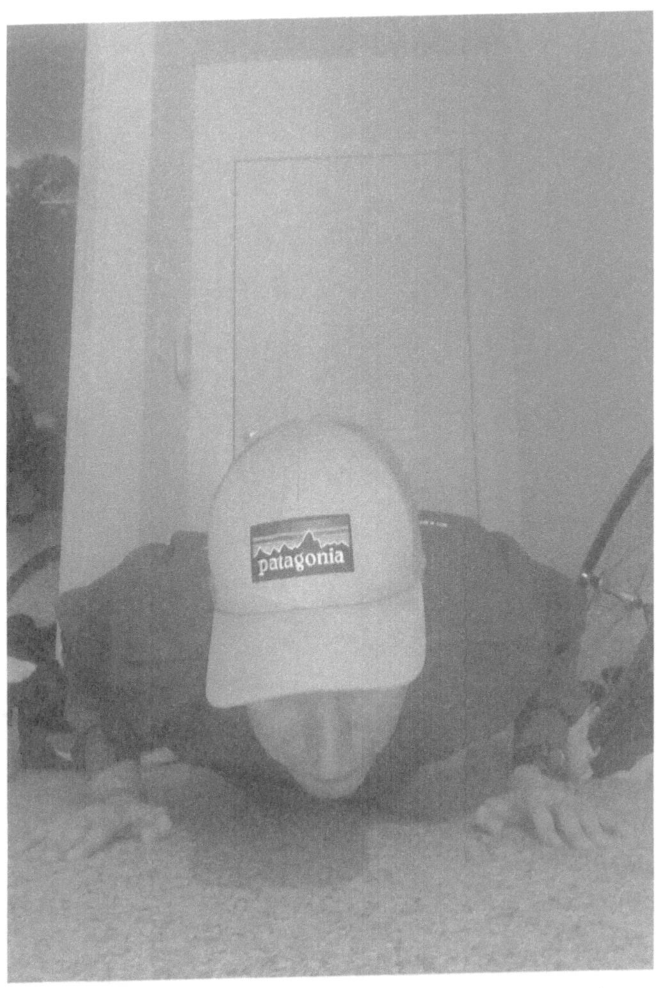

Drop down so chest is almost touching ground

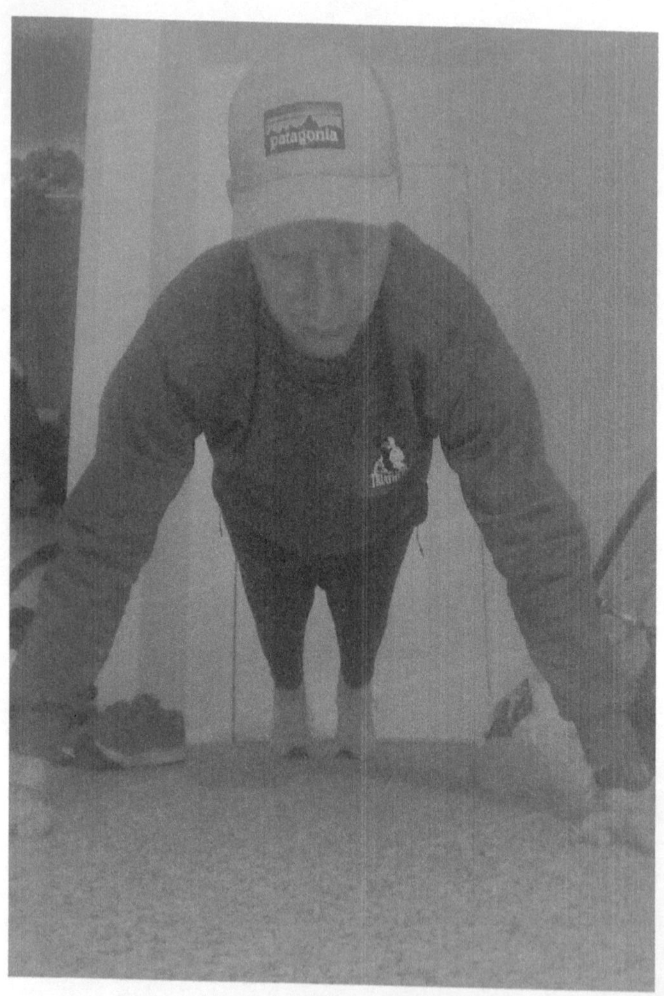

Wide push-up beginning position

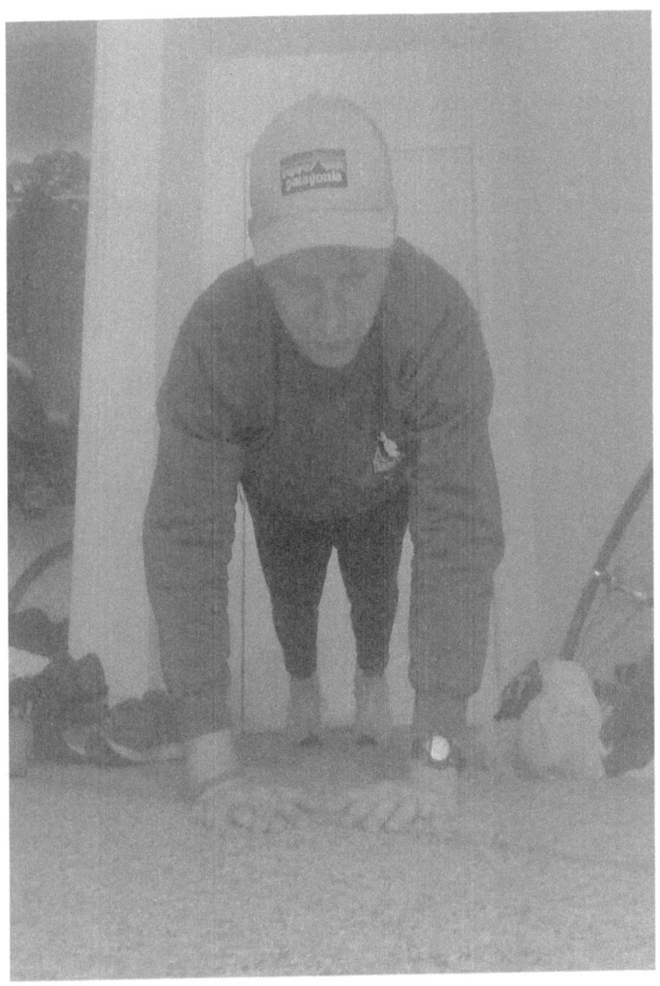

Diamond push-up beginning position

Exercise 4: Step up

The step-up exercise is low-tech and involves either a stair or a step aerobic platform. This exercise works all of your leg muscles and also will get your heart pumping fairly quickly.

To perform the basic step up, simply step up on the platform or stair step like you are walking up a flight of stairs. You want to alternate the leading foot each time so both legs get a balanced workout. Obviously, the steeper the step, the more challenging the exercise is to perform.

- Start standing behind a step.

- Step up onto the platform so both feet are on the top of the platform or stair.

- Lower off the platform by stepping back one foot at a time.

- Repeat, making sure to alternate the leading leg.

Exercise 5: Tricep dip

The tricep dip is a little exercise that works the hard-to-get tricep muscles on the back of your upper arm. It's simple to perform and can be done either with your hands elevated on a bench or chair or with your hands on the ground with you seated. To perform a tricep dip, follow these steps:

- ➢ Place your hands beside your hips, facing forward, either on floor or bench edge.

- ➢ Slide your butt off the bench or raise it up off the floor, so your arms and legs are straight.

- ➢ Lower yourself toward the ground until your elbows are bent back behind you at 90 degrees.

- ➢ Push yourself back up to the starting position and repeat.

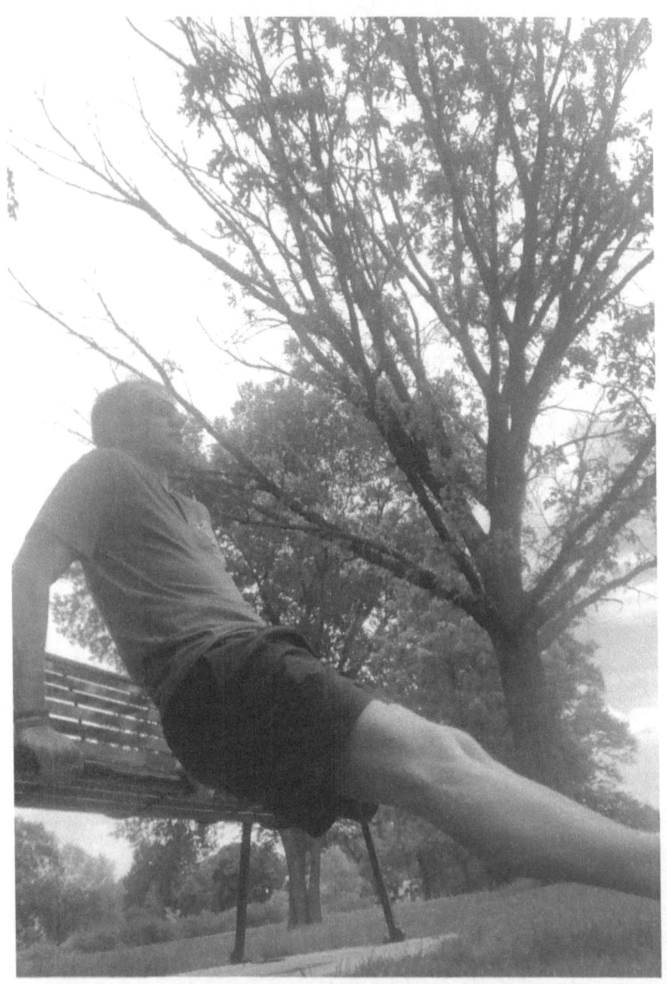

Starting position

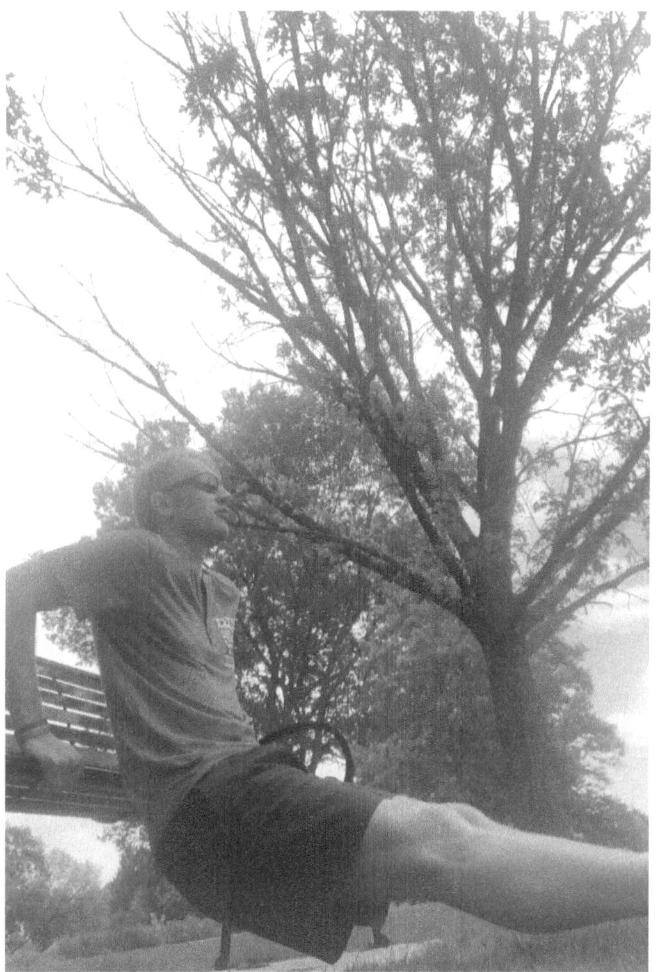

Lower body to ground until elbows bent at 90 degrees.

Exercise 6: Plank

The plank is a great full-body exercise involving your holding a position in place for a fixed period of time—say, 30 seconds or 60 seconds. Performing planks will strengthen your back, abs, shoulders, chest, glutes, quadriceps, and calves.

There are various types of planks, but the most common plank is the forearm plank. Beginners can also start in a push-up position on their hands and toes, arms straight, and hold that until their core and shoulders becomes stronger.

When performing the plank, it is important to keep your back parallel to the ground and your hips/butt level. Then, simply hold that position for the prescribed period of time.

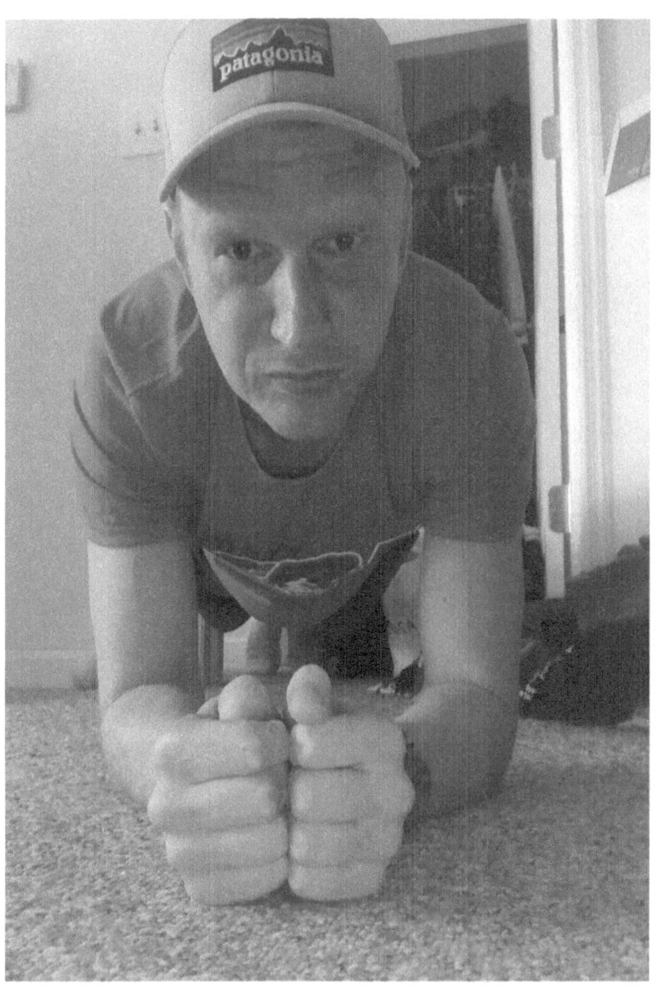

Forearm plank position

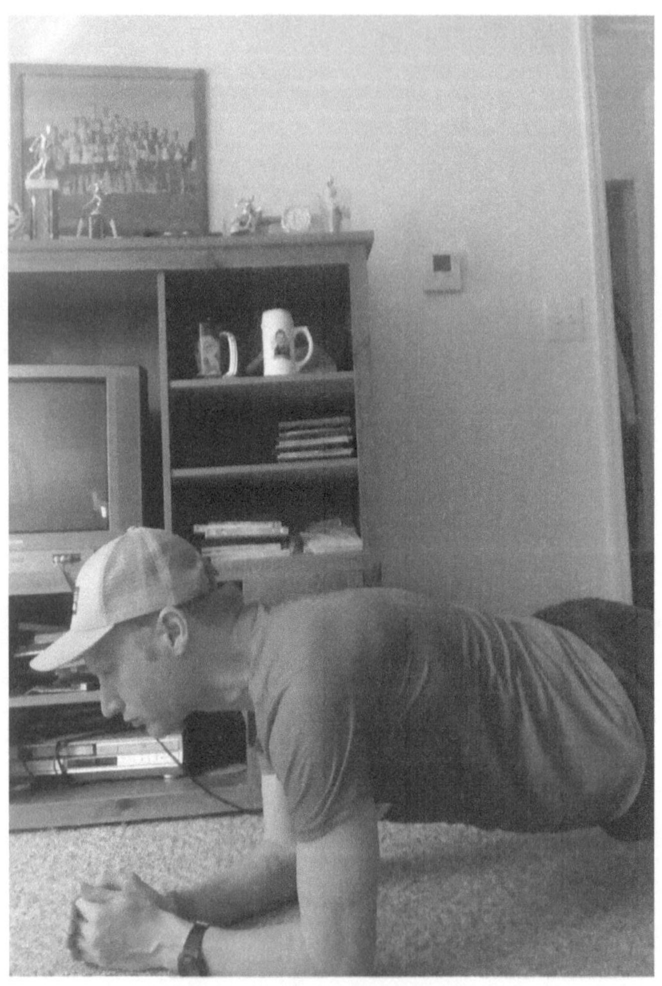

Side view of plank position. Back should be straight!

Exercise 7: High knees

High knees is one of the simples exercises you can do to burn calories and push your heart rate up. You can do high knees at any intensity you want.

To perform high knees, do the following:

➤ Begin in a standing position with your feet together and your arms to your side.

➤ Raise one knee up to a 90-degree position.

➤ Place the foot back down in standing position

➤ Do the same with the other knee.

➤ Repeat the process.

Depending upon your fitness level, you can perform these knee lifts slowly or ramp it up until you are pretty much running in place, using the high-knee form.

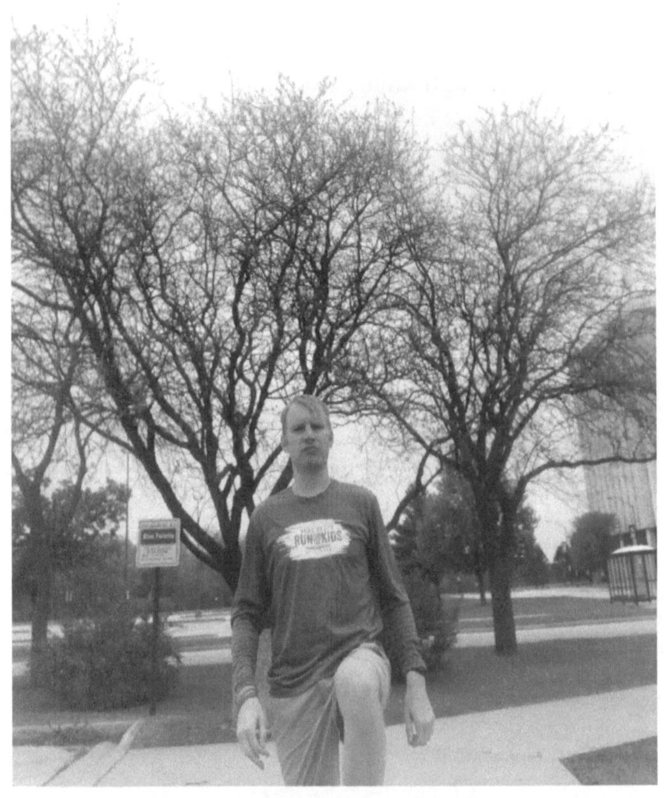

Bring the knee up to 90 degrees

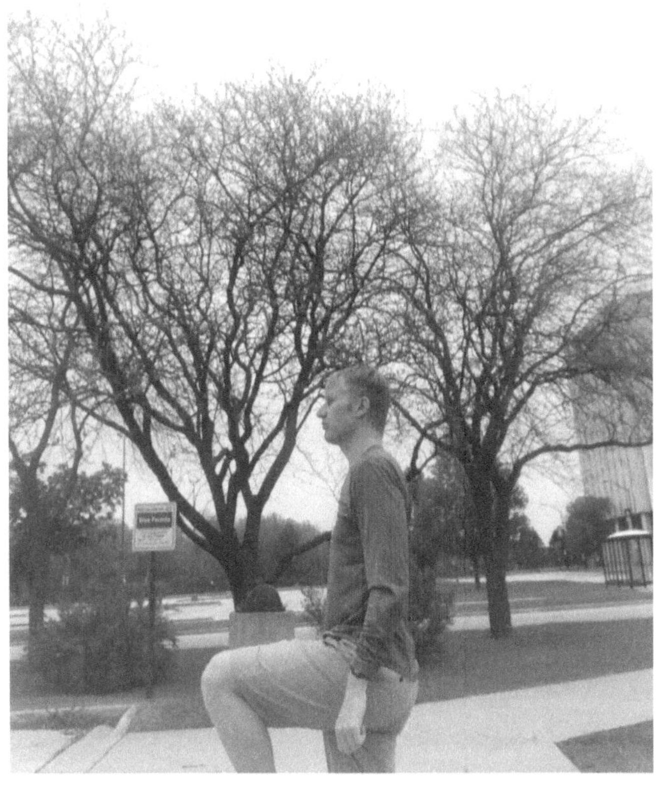

Bring the other knee up to 90 degrees

Exercise 8: Lunges (forward and back)

Lunges are a great exercise to work on your leg and glute muscles. You can do lunges forward, backward, and sideways.

To perform a forward lunge:

➢ Start with your feet together in a standing position.

➢ Take one step forward with your left foot.

➢ Lower your left leg down until your knee bends at 90°, while keeping your right foot planted.

➢ Hold the position for one second and then return back up to the starting position.

➢ Repeat with your right foot and continue to alternate.

A back lunge is the same idea, except you step back with one foot then the other, instead of lunging forward.

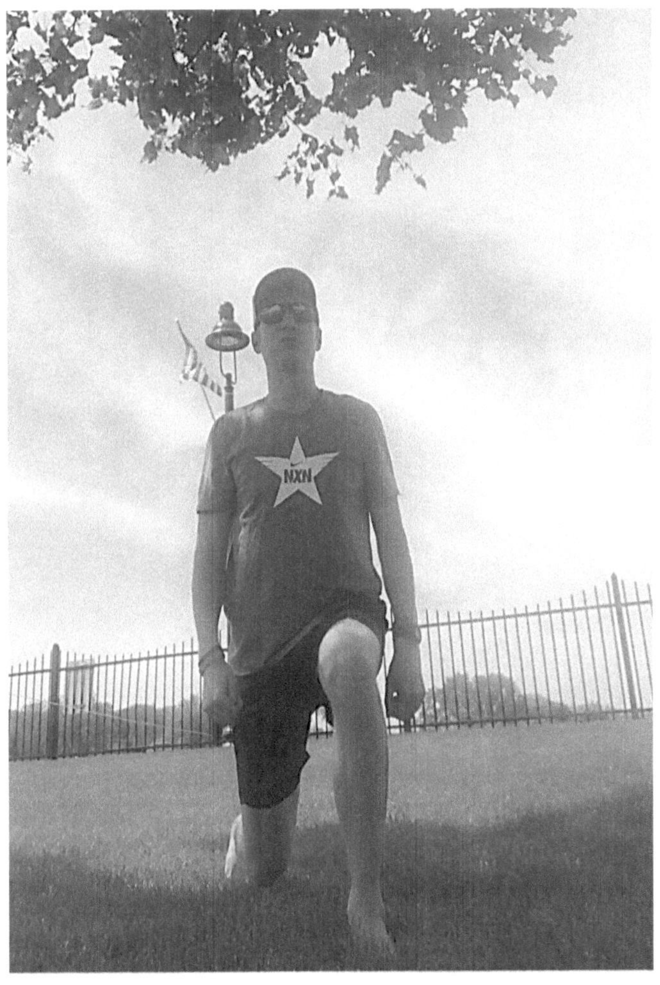
NXN

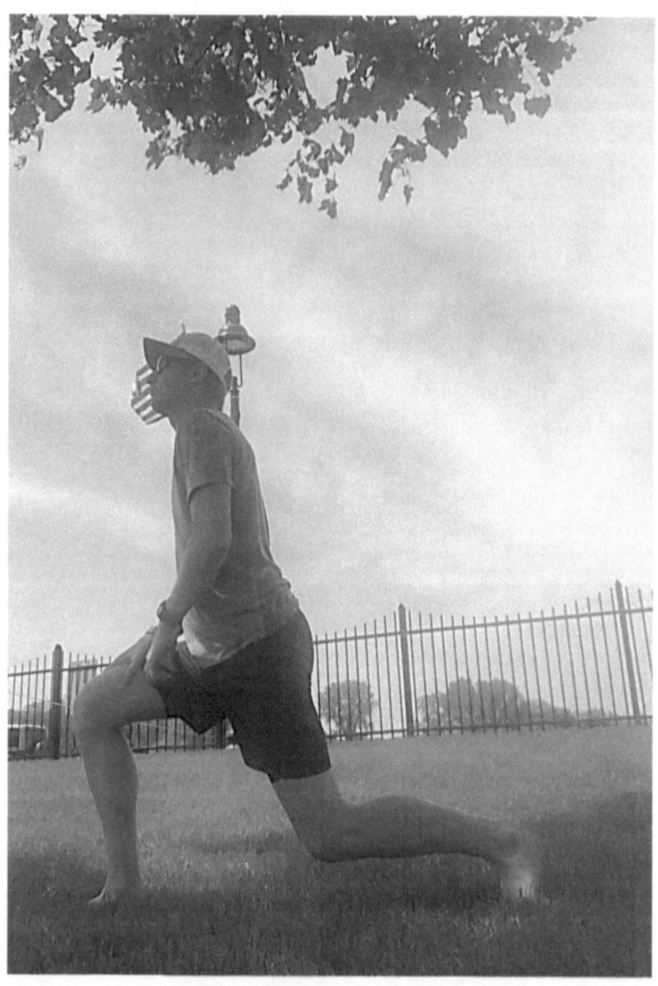

For a complete demonstration of this exercise, check out my Instagram video library: @TheBasicTen

Exercise 9: Jump Rope

Jumping rope is a great way to build lower-leg strength in your calves and feet. It also is a great way to get your heart pumping and lungs working, which leads to burning lots of calories.

In this program, we are actually not going to use a jump rope. Instead, we will pretend we have a jump rope and visualize ourselves jumping over the rope.

For the jump rope exercise, do the following:

➤ Start in a standing position with your feet together.

➤ Pretend you have a jump rope handle in each hand, then simply jump up and down, twisting your wrists, if you like, and visualize yourself jumping over a rope with each leap.

➤ Land on your toes and return to the standing position each time.

Exercise 10: Plank rotations or bicycle crunch

The plank rotations are probably one of the hardest exercises in this program. Plank rotations work your entire core, back, thigh, and glute muscles.

To perform a plank rotation:

➢ Begin in the straight-arm push-up position.

➢ Twist to one side and raise your hand and arm up to the sky (see image). Hold this position for a few seconds.

➢ Return to the starting face-down plank position.

➢ Repeat on the following side.

If you struggle to do plank rotations, do not worry. An alternative exercise is the bicycle crunch. You can modify your plank to start with your knees and calves on the ground.

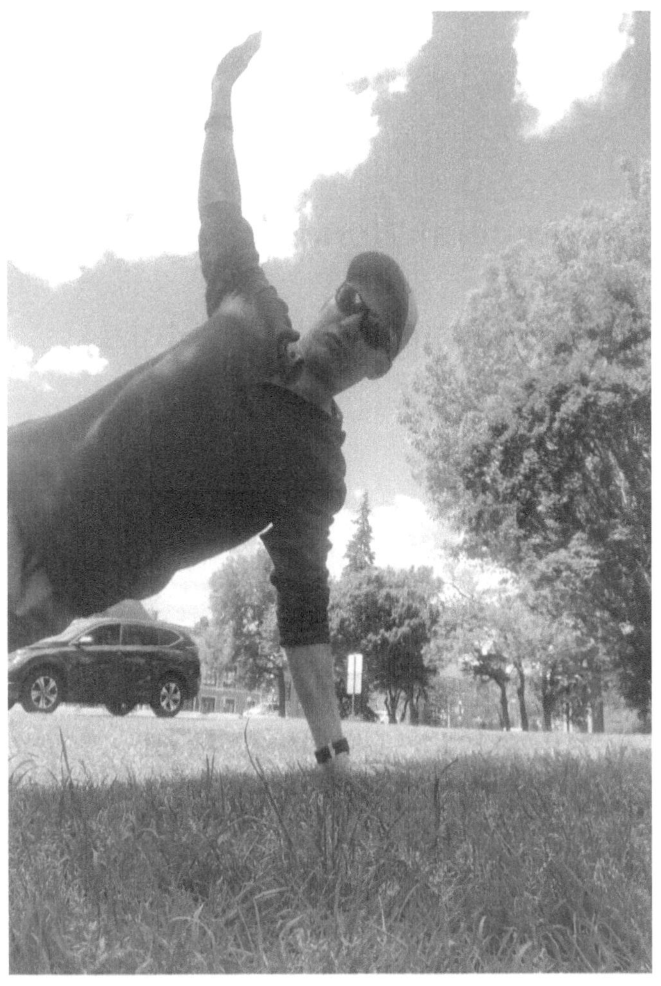

General Workout Design:

Dynamic, Workout, Static

You should always do a dynamic stretch before you begin any actual workout. In the next section, I lay out a specific dynamic routine you can do prior to every workout.

Then, after you finish your workout, take time to do a static stretch. Ahead, I have included another chapter with a static stretching routine you can do after each workout.

So, your daily workout routine should be as follows:

* Dynamic warm up
* Actual listed workout
* Static stretch

Dynamic Warm-up/Stretching

It is a good idea to spend a few minutes doing a short dynamic warm-up before diving into each daily workout. The purpose of a dynamic warm-up is to get the muscles ready for physical activity and to improve their range of motion prior to exercise.

A good dynamic warm-up will reduce your risk of injury and enhance the quality of your workout. It also will improve the connection between your brain and your muscles, something known as the neuromuscular connection.

The following is a simple, easy dynamic warm-up routine you can do. If you go to my Instagram video library: @TheBasicTen, I provide a short demonstration of each exercise.

- ➢ Do each exercise for about twenty seconds.
    - ✓ High knees
    - ✓ Butt kicks
    - ✓ Toe pushes
    - ✓ Back twists
    - ✓ Leg swings to the front
    - ✓ Leg swings to the side

Static Stretching

Static stretching means simply holding a stretch in place for twenty to sixty seconds. By doing so, you will be able to stretch slightly past your comfort zone but not to the point of pain.

Static stretching is a great way to improve your flexibility and reduce your risk of long-term injury.

The best time to do a static stretch is after a workout, when your muscles are nice and warm. The following is a simple static stretching routine. My Instagram video library, @TheBasicTen, has demonstrations of each.

53

- ✓ Hamstrings
- ✓ Quadriceps
- ✓ Calves
- ✓ Hip flexor
- ✓ Back
- ✓ Groin
- ✓ Feet

8-Week Program:

The Layout of the Workouts

There is a total of forty workouts designed for this program. The program is set up so you complete five workouts per week and will be completely done with the program in eight weeks. Some people, however, may want or need to go at a slower pace and complete fewer workouts per week, which is fine. Just pick up with the next workout in the series after a rest day or two and continue through the sequence as you can. You'll still make it to Workout 40!

Do not feel bad if you need to take a day or two off because you feel sore or low on energy. You can do five workouts per week if you feel like it. Or just accomplish two or three per week.

Make sure, however, that you are consistent with the program. Try not to allow yourself to take too many days off, as you are more likely not to return. I would make sure to complete no less than two workouts per week and always more, where possible.

Reminder: Always begin each workout described below with the dynamic warm-up routine and then do the static stretching routine after each workout.

Workout 1

➢ Do a total of 3 rounds of all the listed exercises, in order.

➢ March in place for 20 seconds between each exercise.

✓ 15 Jumping Jacks

✓ 10 squats

✓ 5 push-ups

✓ 20 seconds jumping rope

✓ 5 tricep dips

Workout 2

➢ Do a total of 3 rounds.

➢ March in place for 20 seconds between each exercise.

- ✓ 20 seconds of high knees
- ✓ 20-second plank
- ✓ 20 seconds of step-ups
- ✓ 4 plank rotations
- ✓ 8 lunges (4 on each leg)

Workout 3

➢ Do 3 rounds total.

➢ March in place for 20 seconds to rest between exercises.

- ✓ 20 Jumping Jacks
- ✓ 12 squats
- ✓ 7 push-ups
- ✓ 30 seconds of jump rope
- ✓ 7 tricep dips

Workout 4

- ➤ Do 3 rounds
- ➤ March in place for 20 seconds between each

  - ✓ 30 seconds high knees
  - ✓ 30-second plank
  - ✓ 30 seconds step-ups
  - ✓ 6 plank rotations
  - ✓ 10 lunges

Workout 5

➢ Do 3 rounds total.

➢ Walk in place for 40 seconds between each exercise.

- ✓ 30 seconds or Jumping Jacks
- ✓ 30 seconds high knees
- ✓ 30 seconds jump rope
- ✓ 30 seconds step-ups

###

Congratulations on making it through the first week! Take a few days to recover and celebrate the fact that you made it this far. Remember: the most important part about fitness and health is consistency. Get back strong next week and enjoy the journey.

Workout 6

- ➢ Do 3 rounds

- ➢ March in place for 20 seconds between each exercise

  - ✓ 30 seconds Jumping Jacks
  - ✓ 20 seconds push-ups
  - ✓ 30 seconds jump rope
  - ✓ 20 seconds tricep dips
  - ✓ 30 seconds high knees

Workout 7

➢ Do 3 rounds

➢ March in place for 20 seconds between each exercise

- ✓ 30 seconds jump rope
- ✓ 30-second plank
- ✓ 30 seconds high knees
- ✓ 30 seconds of plank rotation or bicycle crunch
- ✓ 30 seconds Jumping Jacks

Workout 8

- ➢ Complete 3 rounds
- ➢ Walk in place for 20 seconds between each exercise
  - ✓ 30 seconds high knees
  - ✓ 30 seconds step-ups
  - ✓ 30 seconds Jumping Jacks
  - ✓ 30 seconds squats
  - ✓ 30 seconds jump rope
  - ✓ 30 seconds lunges

Workout 9

➢ Complete 1 round only

➢ March in place for 30 seconds between each exercise

✓ 30 seconds jump rope

✓ 20 seconds tricep dips

✓ 30 seconds high knees

✓ 30-second plank

✓ 30 seconds squats

✓ 20 seconds push-ups

✓ 30 second step up

✓ 20 seconds plank rotations

✓ 30 seconds Jumping Jacks

✓ 30 seconds lunges

Workout 10

- ➢ Complete only 1 round.

- ➢ March in place for 30 seconds between each exercise.

  - ✓ 20 seconds jump rope
  - ✓ 20 seconds Jumping Jacks
  - ✓ 20 seconds step-ups
  - ✓ 20 seconds high knees
  - ✓ 40 seconds jump rope
  - ✓ 40 seconds Jumping Jacks
  - ✓ 40 seconds step ups
  - ✓ 40 seconds high knees
  - ✓ 20 seconds jump rope
  - ✓ 20 seconds Jumping Jacks
  - ✓ 20 seconds step ups
  - ✓ 20 seconds high knees

####

Awesome job making it two weeks into the program. Hopefully you are starting to feel a little stronger and more fit. The big thing is consistency and taking time to recover after each workout.

Rest and recover for a few days, so you are ready for another challenging week.

Workout 11

- Complete 4 rounds
- March in place for 20 seconds between each exercise
  - ✓ 20 seconds Jumping Jacks
  - ✓ 20 seconds jump rope
  - ✓ 20 seconds high knees
  - ✓ 20 seconds push-ups
  - ✓ 20 seconds tricep dips

Workout 12

➢ Complete 3 rounds

➢ March in place for 20 seconds between each exercise

- ✓ 40 seconds high knees
- ✓ 35 seconds plank
- ✓ 30 seconds Jumping Jacks
- ✓ 30 seconds plank rotations or bicycle crunch
- ✓ 30 second steps-ups

Workout 13

- ➤ Complete 4 rounds

- ➤ March in place for 20 seconds between each

    - ✓ 30 seconds Jumping Jacks
    - ✓ 30 seconds jump rope
    - ✓ 30 seconds squats
    - ✓ 30 seconds lunges

Workout 14

- ➤ Complete 1 round

- ➤ March in place for 20 seconds between each exercise

  - ✓ 30 seconds jump rope
  - ✓ 30 seconds Jumping Jacks
  - ✓ 30 seconds step ups
  - ✓ 40 seconds high knees
  - ✓ 40 seconds jump rope
  - ✓ 40 seconds Jumping Jacks
  - ✓ 40 seconds step up
  - ✓ 40 seconds high knees
  - ✓ 30 seconds jump rope
  - ✓ 30 seconds Jumping Jacks
  - ✓ 30 seconds step ups
  - ✓ 30 seconds high knees

Workout 15

➢ Complete 1 round

➢ March in place for 20 seconds between each exercise.

✓ 30 seconds jump rope
✓ 30 second Jumping Jacks
✓ 30 seconds step-ups
✓ 30 seconds high knees
✓ 40 seconds jump rope
✓ 40 seconds Jumping Jacks
✓ 40 seconds step up
✓ 40 seconds high knees
✓ 30 seconds jump rope
✓ 30 seconds Jumping Jacks
✓ 30 seconds step-ups
✓ 30 seconds high knees

###

Give yourself a huge pat on the back for completing the first three weeks of the program. Hopefully, you're feeling better physically and mentally. Continue to push yourself and do your best every day.

Enjoy a few off days before getting back on it next week.

Workout 16

- ➢ Complete 3 rounds
- ➢ Do 20 seconds of marching in place between exercises
  - ✓ 30 seconds jump rope
  - ✓ 30 seconds push-ups
  - ✓ 30 seconds Jumping Jacks
  - ✓ 30 seconds tricep dips
  - ✓ 30 seconds knee raises

Workout 17

> Complete 2 rounds
> March in place for 20 seconds between each
>> 30 seconds step-ups
>> 20 seconds plank
>> 30 seconds jump rope
>> 20 seconds plank
>> 30 seconds Jumping Jacks
>> 30 seconds plank rotations or bicycle crunch
>> 30 seconds high knees
>> 40 seconds squats

Workout 18

- ➢ Complete 2 rounds
- ➢ 20 seconds march in place between exercises
  - ✓ 40 seconds Jumping jacks
  - ✓ 40 seconds lunges
  - ✓ 40 seconds high knees
  - ✓ 40 seconds squats
  - ✓ 40 seconds jump rope
  - ✓ 40 seconds step-ups

Workout 19

➢ Complete 1 round

➢ March in place for 20 seconds between exercises

- ✓ 10 seconds jump rope
- ✓ 20 seconds jump rope
- ✓ 30 seconds jump rope
- ✓ 30 seconds push-ups
- ✓ 10 seconds step-ups
- ✓ 20 seconds step-ups
- ✓ 30 seconds step-ups
- ✓ 30 seconds tricep dips
- ✓ 10 seconds Jumping Jack
- ✓ 20 seconds Jumping Jack

- ✓ 30 seconds Jumping Jacks
- ✓ 40 seconds plank
- ✓ 10 seconds high knee
- ✓ 20 seconds high knee
- ✓ 30 seconds high knee

Workout 20

- ➢ Complete 4 rounds
- ➢ 20 seconds march in place between each
  - ✓ 40 seconds Jumping Jacks
  - ✓ 20 seconds plank rotations or bicycle crunch
  - ✓ 40 seconds Jumping Jacks
  - ✓ 20 seconds squats

###

Awesome job! You are exactly halfway through the program. Hopefully, you are seeing the physical and mental benefits from regular physical activity that engages all of your muscle groups.

Celebrate your accomplishment! The rest of the program will be challenging but even more fun.

Workout 21

➢ Complete 3 rounds.

➢ March in place for 20 seconds between each exercise.

- ✓ 40 seconds Jumping Jacks
- ✓ 30 seconds push-ups
- ✓ 40 seconds Jumping Jacks
- ✓ 30 seconds tricep dips
- ✓ 40 seconds Jumping Jacks

Workout 22

- ➤ Complete 3 rounds.

- ➤ March in place for 20 seconds between each.
  - ✓ 40 seconds step-ups
  - ✓ 40 seconds plank
  - ✓ 40 seconds jump rope
  - ✓ 40 seconds squats

Workout 23

➢ Complete 4 rounds.

➢ March in place for 30 seconds between each exercise.

  ✓ 40 seconds high knees
  ✓ 30 seconds plank rotations
  ✓ 40 seconds lunges

Workout 24

> ➤ Complete 4 rounds.

> ➤ March in place for 10 seconds between each exercise.

- ✓ 45 seconds Jumping Jacks
- ✓ 45 seconds squats
- ✓ 45 seconds jump rope
- ✓ 45 seconds high knees

Workout 25

➢ Complete 2 rounds.

➢ March in place 20 seconds between each exercise.

- ✓ 20 seconds push-ups regular style
- ✓ 40 seconds Jumping Jacks
- ✓ 20 seconds push-ups, diamond-style
- ✓ 40 seconds Jumping Jacks
- ✓ 20 seconds push-ups, wide hands
- ✓ 40 seconds Jumping Jacks
- ✓ 20 seconds tricep dips

###

Awesome week of effort. Your body and mind and starting to get stronger.

You have now passed the halfway point of the program. Keep it up and celebrate!

Workout 26

- ➢ Complete 3 rounds.

- ➢ March in place for 20 seconds between each exercise.

  - ✓ 40 seconds jump rope
  - ✓ 40 seconds plank
  - ✓ 40 seconds jump rope
  - ✓ 40 seconds plank rotations

Workout 27

> - Complete 4 rounds.

> - March in place for 20 seconds between each exercise.

  - ✓ 40 seconds squats
  - ✓ 40 seconds lunges
  - ✓ 40 seconds step-ups

Workout 28

- ➤ Complete 3 rounds.

- ➤ March in place for 20 seconds between each exercise.

  - ✓ 40 seconds high knees
  - ✓ 40 seconds Jumping Jacks
  - ✓ 40 seconds jump rope
  - ✓ 40 seconds step-ups

Workout 27

- ➢ Complete 4 rounds.

- ➢ March in place for 20 seconds between each exercise.

  - ✓ 40 seconds squats
  - ✓ 40 seconds lunges
  - ✓ 40 seconds step-ups

Workout 28

> ➢ Complete 3 rounds.

> ➢ March in place for 20 seconds between each exercise.

- ✓ 40 seconds high knees
- ✓ 40 seconds Jumping Jacks
- ✓ 40 seconds jump rope
- ✓ 40 seconds step-ups

Workout 29

- ➢ Compete 1 round only.
- ➢ March in place for 20 seconds between each exercise.
  - ✓ 30 seconds push-ups
  - ✓ 30 seconds planks
  - ✓ 30 seconds squats
  - ✓ 30 seconds wide push-ups
  - ✓ 30 seconds plank rotations or bicycle crunch
  - ✓ 30 seconds lunges
  - ✓ 30 seconds diamond push-ups
  - ✓ 30 seconds plank
  - ✓ 30 second jump rope
  - ✓ 30 seconds high knees
  - ✓ 30 seconds plank rotations or bicycle crunch

Workout 30

- ➤ Complete only 1 round.

- ➤ March in place 10 seconds between each exercise.
  - ✓ 30 seconds jump rope
  - ✓ 30 seconds Jumping Jacks
  - ✓ 30 seconds step-ups
  - ✓ 30 seconds high knees
  - ✓ 40 seconds plank
  - ✓ 30 seconds jump rope
  - ✓ 30 seconds step-ups
  - ✓ 30 seconds high knees
  - ✓ 40 seconds plank rotations or bicycle crunches.

- ✓ 30 seconds jump rope
- ✓ 30 seconds Jumping Jacks
- ✓ 30 seconds step-ups
- ✓ 30 seconds high knees

###

Great job this week. Those workouts were not easy, but you were able to conquer the challenges. The next two weeks will continue to challenge you, but you will persevere, if you set your mind to it.

Take a few days off and start fresh. Just ten more workouts to go. You've got this!

Workout 31

➢ Complete 2 rounds.

➢ March in place for 20 seconds between each exercise.

- ✓ 40 seconds high knees
- ✓ 30 seconds push-ups
- ✓ 40 seconds squats
- ✓ 40 seconds planks
- ✓ 40 seconds Jumping Jacks

Workout 32

> ➢ Complete 4 rounds.

> ➢ March in place 20 seconds between each exercise.

> - ✓ 40 seconds step-ups
> - ✓ 40 seconds plank rotations
> - ✓ 40 seconds jump rope

Workout 33

➢ Compete 3 rounds.

➢ 20 seconds marching in place between each exercise.

✓ 40 seconds Jumping Jacks
✓ 30 seconds tricep dips
✓ 40 seconds lunges
✓ 30 seconds diamond push-ups

Workout 34

> Complete 4 rounds.

> 20 seconds walking in place between each exercise.

- ✓ 1 minute of squats
- ✓ 40 seconds plank
- ✓ 1 minute of high knees (fast-paced)

Workout 35

- ➤ Complete 3 rounds.

- ➤ March in place for 30 seconds between each exercise.

    - ✓ 45 seconds jump rope
    - ✓ 45 seconds step-ups
    - ✓ 45 seconds Jumping Jacks
    - ✓ 45 seconds high knees

Awesome job so far. You should be incredibly proud of yourself for making it this far in the program. Next week will be your last week. Continue to give it all that you have. Way to go!

Workout 36

➢ Complete 3 rounds.

➢ March in place for 15 seconds between each exercise.

- ✓ 40 seconds Jumping Jacks
- ✓ 20 seconds regular push-ups
- ✓ 40 seconds step-ups
- ✓ 20 seconds diamond push-ups
- ✓ 40 seconds jump rope
- ✓ 20 seconds wide push-ups
- ✓ 1 minute of high knees

Workout 37

- ➢ Complete 3 rounds.
- ➢ Walk in place for 10 seconds between each exercise.
  - ✓ 30 seconds Jumping Jacks
  - ✓ 40 seconds squats
  - ✓ 30 seconds Jumping Jacks
  - ✓ 40 seconds lunges
  - ✓ 30 seconds Jumping Jacks
  - ✓ 40 seconds wide squat
  - ✓ 30 seconds Jumping Jacks

Workout 38

- ➢ Complete 3 rounds.
- ➢ Walk in place for 20 seconds between each exercise.
  - ✓ 40 seconds plank rotations
  - ✓ 40 seconds step-ups
  - ✓ 40 seconds planks
  - ✓ 40 seconds jump rope

Workout 39

➢ Complete 3 rounds.

➢ Walk in place for 20 seconds between each exercise.

- ✓ 40 seconds push-ups
- ✓ 40 seconds squats
- ✓ 40 seconds Jumping Jacks
- ✓ 40 seconds tricep dips
- ✓ 40 seconds jump rope

Workout 40

- ➢ Complete 3 rounds.
- ➢ 15 seconds marching in place between exercise.
  - ✓ 30 seconds step-ups
  - ✓ 30 seconds squats
  - ✓ 30 seconds Jumping Jacks
  - ✓ 30 seconds lunges
  - ✓ 30 seconds jump rope
  - ✓ 30 seconds high knees

Nutrition Tips

If you're looking to maximize the benefit you get from this program, you will want to consume a healthy diet. Most likely you will find yourself motivated to eat more fresh, nutritious food now that you have taken on an exercise program.

When it comes to nutrition, think about a diet of more fruits and vegetables and less of everything else. Aim for as many different colors of fruits and vegetables as you possibly can every day. With every meal you consume, at least half of your plate should consist of plant-based foods.

Enjoy your favorite foods and treats in moderation. In particular, watch your consumption of sugary drinks and alcoholic beverages. These provide a lot of calories and do not nourish our bodies at all.

General Health Tips

Everything in moderation! There's a lot of truth to this simple saying. Our eating habits and fitness routines do not need to be perfect, but we do need to make sure to keep everything in balance. We need to eat healthy, nutrient-dense, preferably plant-based foods most of the time and continue to get some form of regular physical activity.

You do not need to be perfect with your fitness and exercise routine. If you take a few days off now and then, you will bounce back just fine, when you resume. That said, it is important to keep up with your exercise program on a regular basis and not let yourself remain idle for too long.

When it comes to exercise and physical activity, **consistency** is the main thing. People who are successful with their nutrition and exercise are those who do it on a consistent basis. They find the time and the place to get in their workout each day.

Going hard for a period of time and then doing nothing for several weeks is going to be less effective than doing simple, easy workouts regularly. Regular and consistent exercise will give you the best physical and mental benefits.

What's Next, After You Master These Workouts

Congratulations! You have successfully completed the program. You now should be stronger and fitter than before. You definitely should take some time to celebrate your accomplishment. It is very important to take a moment to acknowledge the work you have done and the progress you've made.

You may begin to wonder what you should do next in terms of your workout routine and physical activity. I would encourage you to take on another challenge, whether it be doing the program again and adding more repetitions of each exercise, or starting a new program.

Or perhaps you were looking to do something different, such as train for a 5K road race or maybe bike 100 miles. Whatever the next thing is in your journey, you are now more prepared.

You could also use the exercises in this program to design your own workouts or repeat the current workouts adding more repetitions or time for each one.

Check back frequently with my Instagram video library, @TheBasicTen, as I may add another, more advanced program that you can try out. As always, feel free to reach out to me, if you have any questions or comments on the program.

Good luck and stay strong!

Ben Mueller

Email: Ben.mueller7@aol.com

All demo videos on Instagram: @TheBasicTen

Author Note

Reviews, recommendations, and shares are incredibly valuable to authors. If you enjoyed this program, please consider sharing it with others by:

> ➤ Leaving a rating and review of *The Basic Ten* on mazon.com.
>
> ➤ Joining and following the Basic Ten Instagram fan page: @TheBasicTen.
>
> ➤ Telling your family and friends about the program, if they could benefit from it.

Thank you!

About Ben Mueller

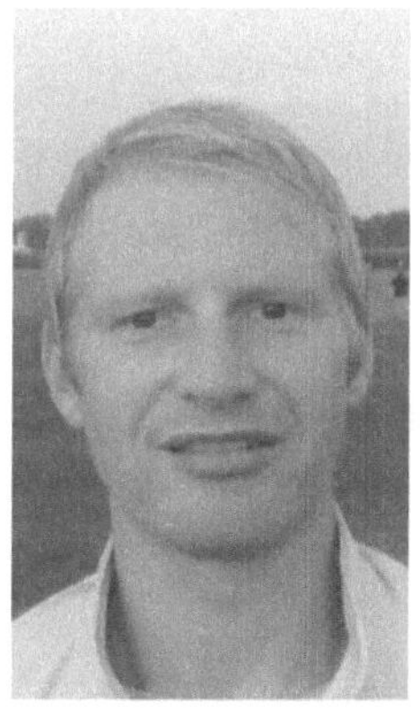

Ben Mueller is a wellness educator, endurance athlete, speaker, and activist. He has taught high school and junior college health and mathematics for over fifteen years.

Since he completed his first road race at the age of ten, Ben has not looked back. He is an avid runner and triathlete who has competed in over 500 road races, track races, and triathlons throughout the United States.

He qualified and competed in the United States national triathlon championships three times. He is also a Badger State Games (Wisconsin Olympics) gold medalist for multiple years in both the open and Masters categories.

Ben was born in Sheboygan, Wisconsin and went to college at UW-Whitewater. He earned his bachelor's degree in mathematics education and a master's degree in educational leadership at Concordia-Chicago. Currently, he is a doctoral student in education at Concordia-Chicago, doing his PhD research on exercise and its effects on coping with math anxiety.

When Ben is not training, he can be found refereeing soccer, rooting on the Wisconsin sports teams, or relaxing in a coffee shop.

Contact Ben here: Ben.mueller7@aol.com

Or find him here: BenjaminTMueller.webs.com

Also by Ben Mueller

Attain Peak Running Through Cross-Training

Attain Peak Referee Fitness

The Operating Manual for Great Health

30 Minutes to Peak Thinking